D1799466

HowExpert Presents

How to Live with PCOS

HowExpert with Melissa Hayden

Copyright HowExpert™
www.HowExpert.com

For more tips related to this topic, visit HowExpert.com/pcos.

Recommended Resources

- HowExpert.com – Quick 'How To' Guides on All Topics from A to Z by Everyday Experts.
- HowExpert.com/free – Free HowExpert Email Newsletter.
- HowExpert.com/books – HowExpert Books
- HowExpert.com/courses – HowExpert Courses
- HowExpert.com/clothing – HowExpert Clothing
- HowExpert.com/membership – HowExpert Membership Site
- HowExpert.com/affiliates – HowExpert Affiliate Program
- HowExpert.com/writers – Write About Your #1 Passion/Knowledge/Expertise & Become a HowExpert Author.
- HowExpert.com/resources – Additional HowExpert Recommended Resources
- YouTube.com/HowExpert – Subscribe to HowExpert YouTube.
- Instagram.com/HowExpert – Follow HowExpert on Instagram.
- Facebook.com/HowExpert – Follow HowExpert on Facebook.

Table of Contents

Introduction

Polycystic ovary syndrome, also known as PCOS, is a relatively new diagnosis in the world of medicine. The first description of it was made in 1935, but only since the start of the 21st century have doctors started to really understand the causes, effects, and most effective treatments for PCOS. And even now, a ridiculous number of doctors seem to have no clue how to really treat it!

By some estimates, as many as 10% of the world's women may suffer from polycystic ovary syndrome. That's a lot of women! Yet, many of these women know little about the condition itself – what it is, what it can mean for them, and most importantly, how to treat it.

If you have been diagnosed with PCOS, it can feel overwhelming. Often times, a general practitioner or primary care doctor will give the diagnosis, but will not understand much about how the woman can best live with this incurable condition. Sadly, many times doctors will prescribe "standard" treatments (usually either birth control pills, metformin, or a combination), but will do little else.

If this is the situation you are in; don't worry—you are not alone! This guide will help you learn, in 7 steps, how to best control your PCOS. Your goal should not be to simply grin and bear it, but to learn how you can have a happy and fulfilling life while living with PCOS.

Please remember that this is not a medical textbook or guide; the information here is based on personal experience living with PCOS, and is not a replacement for seeking proper medical care. See section 2 for help learning how to find a good doctor who can assist with your individual health care needs.

Step 1: Know Your Enemy (By Learning About PCOS)

You sit in a chilly, white-walled room, dressed only in an awkward paper gown. You've just been through a battery of tests, and feel anxious to hear the doctor's diagnosis. After what feels like an eternity, the doctor steps into the room, silently reviewing your file as he sits. In a matter of fact tone, he says four simple words which will change your life forever. "You have PCOS."

If you have heard those words, you know how upsetting they can be. Receiving a diagnosis of polycystic ovary syndrome is not like receiving a diagnosis of cancer. When a doctor tells you that you have cancer, they are sympathetic, consoling, and full of information – what does this mean for you; what does your future look like; what are your treatment options? Far too often, when a woman is told she has PCOS, it is not done with any sympathy or consoling, and rarely is the doctor ready with information. That's why, when talking about how to live with PCOS, the first thing most women need to do is to take it upon themselves to learn more about polycystic ovary syndrome. Here, we will provide an overview of what PCOS is, what are its causes, and how it affects women over the course of their lives.

Remember 6th Grade Health Class?

To understand PCOS, first you must understand how the menstrual cycle works. For those who don't remember the awkward slide-shows and videos from health class, here's the (very simplified) breakdown.

First, **estrogen and progesterone** levels start to rise. This does a lot for a woman's body, but one important effect is that the increase in hormones triggers a thickening in the lining of the uterus. This is the body preparing to host a fertilized embryo.

Next, during ovulation, a mature egg leaves the ovary and travel through the fallopian tubes to the uterus. If the egg has not been fertilized when it reaches the uterus, hormone levels drop, causing menstruation (a shedding of the egg and uterine lining).

So, the take away from this is that hormones are the catalyst for everything in the menstrual cycle, and if they are not in balance or if something disrupts the production of estrogen, progesterone, or other hormones (like **Leutenizing Hormone** or **Follicle Stimulating Hormone**), then menstruation may not take place.

PCOS Messes Up Hormones

PCOS does not look the same for every woman. There are a list of symptoms which doctors use to diagnose the condition, but not all women will have every symptom. There are a variety of tests which might (or might not!) be used to diagnose PCOS. What all cases do have in common though is this: *the patient's hormone levels are out of balance.* That's the real definition of PCOS, no matter what long-winded speeches a doctor might give.

PCOS is indicated by a disruption in the hormonal balance of a woman's body. Because hormones are so vital to the menstrual cycle, this means that most women with PCOS experience irregular or absent periods, as well as infertility.

The name of the condition, polycystic ovary syndrome, seems to indicate that it is caused by multiple cysts on the ovaries—that would make sense, right? In reality, PCOS *causes* cysts to form on the ovaries (of some women), but that's not what causes the condition. If it were, it would be easy to cure by removing the cysts surgically. But truthfully, doctors don't know what causes PCOS, and many women are diagnosed without having any ovarian cysts appear on imaging tests. Doctors believe genetics can play a role, since women are more likely to develop PCOS if their mother or sister has it.

Symptoms and Risk Factors of PCOS

Since PCOS can have many faces, how do you identify it? In a clinic, the two symptoms that are considered the biggest indicators of PCOS are **oligomenorrhea** (irregular periods) and **hyperandrogenism** (an excess of the hormone **androgen**). If you have one or both of these, you will likely be told you have PCOS. Other symptoms may include:

- amenorrhea (absence of periods)
- obesity
- insulin resistance
- obstructive sleep apnea
- hirsutism (excessive hair growth, especially on the face)
- balding or thinning of the hair on the head
- acne

As mentioned, these symptoms may not appear in all women. Many women with PCOS are very thin (this is sometimes called "Lean PCOS"), while others may not experience a significant disruption in their menstrual cycle. Still others have regular periods, but they are extremely painful and heavy. It all depends on what hormones have been affected, and how much your hormone levels are "off."

The symptoms above are what most people imagine when they think of polycystic ovary syndrome, but they are, in effect, the tip of the iceberg. Below the water, PCOS can involve many other risk factors. Women with untreated PCOS are more likely to develop:

- diabetes
- high blood pressure
- high cholesterol
- endometrial cancer
- infertility
- mental health problems (such as depression and anxiety)

- liver disease
- heart attack

With all these risk factors, it is easy to see that PCOS should not be ignored or taken lightly. Learning as much as possible about PCOS is an important first step in successfully living with the condition, because it helps motivate you to action. Committing to and following through with a treatment plan is vital, but you can't do those things if you aren't motivated. So spend some time pondering over your condition, and really think about what the consequences of ignoring it will be for you and your loved ones. Make a list of all the reasons why you are determined to manage your PCOS, and keep it somewhere nearby where you can read it on days when you need an extra shot of motivation.

And when you've mustered up enough motivation, you can move on the next step, which involves assembling a team of physicians.

Step 2: Find the Right Doctor (or Doctors)

It's sad, but true – a good doctor, with knowledge about PCOS, is hard to find. Many times, a primary care physician will diagnose the syndrome, but will not have the experience to be truly helpful in outlining a personalized care plan. There are exceptions, of course; some primary care physicians or nurse practitioners take a special interest in women's health, and will be very knowledgeable. But in most cases, a referral to a specialist is likely warranted.

Finding a Specialist

You might wonder, what kind of specialist should I go to? There are two types of doctor who might specialize in polycystic ovary syndrome. One is an endocrinologist (a doctor who deals with glands and hormones), and the other is a gynecologist (a doctor who deals with the female reproductive system). Which you choose will likely depend on your particular symptoms, as well as the availability of doctors in your area. You may even want to see both; the endocrinologist and gynecologist can work together to share information and create a more comprehensive treatment plan for you. Regardless of the type of doctor you see, you'll probably spend some time picking out the right person.

Picking a doctor can be stressful; you want someone who is knowledgeable, empathetic, and proactive, but it is hard decipher those qualities without actually meeting them in person. The best way to find a good doctor is usually to simply ask around. If you know anyone else who is dealing with PCOS, start by asking them for a recommendation. If you don't know anyone locally who has PCOS, ask your other doctors for a referral. Or, ask friends for a recommendation of a gynecologist, and start researching doctors from there.

Whether you decide to see a general practitioner, endocrinologist, or a gynecologist, the most important thing to remember is this: **find a doctor who specializes or "has a special interest in" polycystic ovary syndrome**. Check the clinic's website, or call and ask the reception staff about this. Not all endocrinologists or gynecologists have the same level of knowledge about this condition, and it is well worth the time and effort needed to find a real "PCOS specialist."

How to Speak Doctor

Sometimes talking to a doctor can feel like the two of you are speaking different languages. Once you have found a specialist and set up an appointment, how can you make sure to communicate effectively with your doctor?

Prepare ahead of time for your appointment by writing down symptoms or medication side effects that you want to mention to the doctor; it's easy to forget these things when you're in that paper gown, under inquisition in the freezing exam room.

Think about the questions you want to ask your doctor, and write those down as well. Bring these notes with you, and make sure to bring a pen so you can jot down any answers or information the doctor has for you.

Be clear in expressing what you expect from treatment (see step 3 of this guide for more information on how to set goals and priorities for treatment). It is easy to be intimidated by doctors, especially when they talk with such authority, but remember that you are in charge of your body, and you need to feel comfortable with whatever medication or treatment is decided on.

Fertility is often the assumed priority for women with PCOS. Maybe that is your top concern, but if not, feel free to speak up and let the doctor know exactly what you are concerned about.

Sometimes, doctors can seem in a hurry to get rid of you; they get behind in their schedule, and need to catch up, or they simply feel stressed and it leads to rushing through appointments. Be your own advocate, and speak up if you don't understand something that the doctor has just said. But be discerning and polite, as well. If you bombard the doctor with questions as soon as they enter the room, they will become frustrated and it may end up wasting even more time. On the other hand, if you listen to the doctor first and save your questions until the end, you might discover that most of your concerns are answered during the visit.

Understand Common Medical Terms Related to PCOS

Learning common PCOS-related terminology will also help your doctor's appointments to go more smoothly. Rather then your doctor spending time explaining these terms, you can focus on discussing your recent symptoms and changes. Below is a list of common words and phrases you may hear associated with PCOS.

Amenorrhea – Absent periods (more than three missed periods in a row)

BMI – Body Mass Index, a way of measuring weight proportions; BMI is found by dividing your weight in kilograms by the square of your height in meters (kg/m2); a BMI of less than 18.5 is considered underweight, over 25 is considered overweight, and over 30 is considered obese

DHEA (Dehydroepiandrosterone) – A hormone which aids in the production of androgen and estrogen, typically higher in women with PCOS; normal levels for women are between 35-430 ug/dl

Electrolysis – A form of permanent hair removal, often considered a treatment for hirsutism

Endometrium – The lining of the uterus which thickens and is shed throughout the menstrual cycle; endometrial cancer is a cancer affecting this lining, which is more likely when a woman does not have regular periods to shed the endometrium

Glycemic Index (GI) and Glycemic Load (GL) – GI is a scale from 0-100 of how fast a food will increase blood glucose levels, and GL is an indication of how much glucose the food will deliver; these are often important factors to consider due to PCOS' role in insulin resistance and high glucose levels; foods with lower GI and GL are better for those with insulin and glucose problems

Hirsutism – Excessive hair growth on the face or body

Insulin Resistance – A condition where insulin is less effective at controlling blood sugar, leading to high blood sugar levels; if untreated, insulin resistance may lead to Type 2 Diabetes

LH (Lutenizing Hormone) – A hormone that helps regulate ovulation, which is typically higher in women with PCOS; normal levels of LH can range from 1.68 IU/L to 16.3 IU/L depending on the time of month testing takes place

Metformin – A medication used to treat Type 2 Diabetes, but which is also commonly used to treat PCOS because controlling blood glucose levels (blood sugar) has been shown to lower testosterone

Oligomenorrhea – Irregular periods

Oral Contraceptives (Birth Control Pills) – A hormone-based pill that is usually used to prevent pregnancy, but is often given to women with PCOS to regulate menstruation; birth control pills do not affect ovulation, so the periods caused by this treatment are sometimes called "false periods"

Sleep Apnea – A condition where breathing stops for brief periods during sleep; common in women with PCOS because of its link with obesity

Stein-Leventhal Syndrome – The original name for PCOS, rarely used in modern times, but you may hear it thrown around by some doctors

String of Pearls – A common term for the appearance of poly-cystic ovaries on imaging exams

Testosterone – A hormone typically considered the male sex hormone, but which is present in all women in small amounts; free testosterone refers to the amount of testosterone active in your body, while total testosterone includes all testosterone present; both free and total testosterone are typically higher in women with PCOS

To learn even more of the lingo around PCOS, see the glossary at the end of this book.

It's important to set up your "team" of doctors and learn how to talk to them early on, because they will be your main resource as questions come up. The next section will talk about planning your priorities and goals, and as we will see, having a good doctor will be invaluable when charting your course.

Step 3: Know Where You're Going (and Write it Down)

What bothers you the most about having PCOS? If you can answer that question, you can start setting the goals and priorities that will guide your treatment plan. Set aside some time to sit quietly by yourself and think about what you want from life, how your PCOS could be a roadblock, and plan a detour route to achieving your goals. A simple example is this: *I want to have children some day. I know that PCOS can cause infertility or make it difficult to conceive. I need to talk to my doctor about how to improve my fertility.* If sitting down and writing out goals like this sounds difficult, try taking it step by step.

List Ways PCOS Affects You

You are unique, and your PCOS is unique. No book, website, or doctor can tell you exactly what your life will be like when you have PCOS. So start by listing how PCOS affects you – be specific and be personal. Here are some examples of things you might list:

- I never know when I might start my period
- I have insulin resistance, but am underweight, and it is hard to follow a diet without losing more weight
- I can't seem to lose weight even when I limit my calories
- I hate having to wax my lip/chin so often!

- I'm worried about my risk for cancer/diabetes/heart attack

There are no wrong answers here, so don't worry about feeling silly over some of the things you write down.

Pick Your Top Three Concerns

After you have written down everything that concerns you about your PCOS, take a good look at the list, and write a number next to each item, starting at one for the item that is most important to you. It may help to re-write the list in order. Then, after each item, jot down a note about why it is important to you. So, for the examples above, you might write something like:

- I never know when I might start my period (That's really inconvenient and has led to some embarrassing moments)
- I have insulin resistance, but am underweight, and it is hard to follow a diet without losing more weight (I know I need to control my blood sugar, but I'm worried about being too thin or not having enough energy to get through the day)
- I can't seem to lose weight even when I limit my calories (I don't feel good about myself and it's hard to be active because I'm overweight)
- I hate having to wax my lip/chin so often! (It's inconvenient and I am self-conscious about the hair)

- I'm worried about my risk for cancer/diabetes/heart attack (I want to stay healthy so I can have a long and happy life)

Again, this is all about figuring out what *your* priorities and goals are, so there are no wrong answers!

Make a Plan

Finally, for each item, write out what you can do about the problem. Many times, that plan might simply be "talk to my doctor about treatment options," which is more than okay! Talking with your doctor should be the first step for anything PCOS-related, even if it seems superficial, or like it doesn't directly relate to your overall health. Hirsutism, for instance, is something that some women hesitate to talk to their doctors about, but there are actually several medications and topical creams that can be prescribed to help slow down this hair growth. If you can't think of any other solution to the problem, then write down "talk to my doctor," because, if you spent the time to find a doctor knowledgeable in PCOS, they will be your best resource for answers.

If you are overwhelmed by the number of items on your list, highlight just the top three items, and focus on those first. As you continue learning more about your condition and putting different treatments into practice, you can revisit your list from time to time and see if you are ready to tackle another problem. Many problems may even be inter-related, and treating one issue can end up resolving another one at the same time. For example, diet and exercise are two of the most popular treatments for polycystic ovary syndrome, because they can help with a wide range of issues. That's why the next two sections will be devoted to these two pillars of PCOS treatment.

Step 4: Let Your Food Fight For You

You should never start a diet or exercise program without talking to your doctor first.

Once more, with feeling – **always talk to your doctor before starting any diet or exercise plan**.

That being said, there are many foods shown by either scientific or anecdotal evidence to fight the symptoms of polycystic ovary syndrome. There are also many foods that should be avoided or used only in moderation. The majority of the information in this section has come from pcosnutrition.com, which is a great resource for questions relating to the effect of different foods on women with PCOS. That website, like this book, are for informational purposes only and are not a substitute for talking to your doctor about your personal nutrition needs.

Foods to Avoid if You Have PCOS

If you have PCOS, you very likely have high insulin levels (this can be confirmed by a blood test done at your primary care doctor's office). Because of this, it is wise to **avoid refined carbohydrates**, which are found in foods such as bread, pasta, rice, chips, candy, and soda. Even whole wheat products have a huge amount of carbs and can dramatically affect your GL, so be conscious of these foods as well.

Milk is filled with hormones – it is meant to help baby cows grow, after all. Androgen (which helps produce testosterone) is highly present in all dairy products, but low-fat and fat-free milk are the worst offenders. It is advisable for women with PCOS to **limit their dairy intake to no more than two servings per day**. More than this could aggravate hyperandrogenism by raising your testosterone levels. Milk can also lead to acne, so if you're trying to clear up your skin, try going dairy-free for a few weeks to see if it helps.

Inflammatory foods are another category that should be limited. Chronic inflammation is very common in women with PCOS. This inflammation can stimulate excess androgen production. A lot of these foods are the same as ones already mentioned, such as refined carbohydrates, soda, and fried foods. **Red meat and processed meats** are also inflammatory and should be avoided.

Learn to Love These Good-For-You Foods

Anti-Inflammatory foods are some of the best for PCOS. They include **tomatoes, olive oil, nuts, and fish,** as well as many types of fruits and vegetables. Many websites online offer comprehensive anti-inflammatory diet plans. But there are other food choices that can help women with PCOS, too.

Processed soy products (like soy milk, hydrogenated soybean oil, and soy protein isolate) have been proven in medical research to have health risks for women with PCOS. However, **unprocessed soy** has actually been shown to have many health benefits, including increasing fertility among women with PCOS. Unprocessed soy products include tofu, edamame, soy nuts, and some brands of soy sauce.

Another great staple of the PCOS diet is the **egg**. Protein is important for women with PCOS, and eggs are chock full of that nutrient, as well as other vitamins and minerals that help keep you healthy and energized. Other sources of protein can help improve fertility, such as **beans, nuts, and legumes**.

Cinnamon is a surprisingly useful spice for women with PCOS. 1.5g per day of cinnamon helped women in a controlled study to have more menstrual cycles (though fertility and ovulation weren't mentioned specifically). Other studies have concluded that cinnamon can help lower fasting glucose levels and lower cholesterol. You can get cinnamon cassia extract as a supplement pill, but because cinnamon has no calories or carbohydrates, you should also feel free to sprinkle it on your meals, snacks, and even coffee.

Lastly, consider swapping out sugary sodas and juices for tea instead. **Spearmint tea** can reduce androgen and help slow down unwanted hair growth. **Green tea** is anti-inflammatory. **Tava tea** is supposed to help boost metabolism as well as reduce insulin levels. And there are many other teas that have great flavor and can help cut cravings for more sugary treats.

Find the Right Balance

When trying to lose weight, most people concern themselves with counting calories, but there are three other major factors to be aware of: fat, carbohydrates, and protein. Having a diet with the proper balance of these three nutrients is important to a woman's health and weight, especially if she has PCOS.

According to one study, published in *The American Journal of Clinical Nutrition,* women with PCOS did best on a diet consisting of:

- 40% calories from lean protein
- 30% calories from good fats (that's low-saturated fat foods, monounsaturated fats, and omega-3 fatty acid foods)

According to the study, this combination tended to improve weight loss and glucose metabolism *without the women restricting the total number of calories consumed*. Eat more and still lose weight? Sounds like a dream come true! Of course, this may not work for everyone, but it is definitely worth a shot if you are having trouble losing weight while counting calories.

The 40/30 rule doesn't have to be followed strictly to see benefits; simply lowering carbohydrate intake can be enough to help shed extra pounds and regulate insulin and other hormones. Some nutritionists recommend eating around 100g carbohydrates per day, while others go as low as 50g. Just be aware that if you have too few carbohydrates, you may feel like you lack the energy to get through the day; so if you start a diet and feel extra fatigued, try increasing your carb intake a few grams at a time until you find the perfect balance for you.

Step 5: Step Up to a Good Exercise Routine

Nutrition is only one piece of the PCOS puzzle. Whether your goal is to lose weight, lower insulin resistance, or just feel better overall, exercise is an important cornerstone of any PCOS treatment plan. Even so, many women hesitate to start exercising because, frankly, it can be overwhelming. What kind of workout is best? How long should it be? What if I can only make it half way through the routine? There are a lot of questions, and most of them can be answered with one simple answer: **it doesn't matter**.

Any exercise is better than no exercise. If you can only manage a 10 or 15 minute walk, start with that. If you hate strength training, then do something aerobic instead. As long as you are doing something (and your doctor approves, of course), you are doing well.

If, however, you are the sort of person who needs a more detailed plan, then here is what the research says about the best exercise for PCOS.

How to Exercise When You Have PCOS

There are limited studies available that specifically look at PCOS and exercise. However, from what's available, strength training (or resistance training) seems to be a great choice because it can help increase insulin sensitivity as well as boost resting metabolic rate. And while PCOS-related research is rare, there is a mountain of information available for people with type-2 diabetes. Since many women with PCOS have similar metabolic issues to those caused by diabetes, it can be useful to research suggestions for diabetic patients. In one study, doctors suggested that diabetic patients participate in at least 150 minutes of moderate-intensity exercise per week, with resistance training three times per week and aerobics two times per week.

Yes, aerobic workouts (or "cardio") are important too, although most women with PCOS don't find a lot of success with straight cardio workouts. That is, it doesn't have as much effect on weight loss, insulin resistance, or muscle growth as resistance training does.

HIIT (High Intensity Interval Training), though, is a form of aerobic exercise that can actually lower insulin resistance better than continuous resistance training. The basic idea of HIIT is that you work with high intensity for brief periods of time, alternating with brief rests. There are different styles of HIIT, including Tabata (an incredibly intense four-minute workout) and Gibala (the beginner version takes about 20 minutes total and calls for 60-second bursts of activity followed by 60 seconds of rest). HIIT is a great way to incorporate cardio into your exercise routine, especially if you're short on time.

While many people use HIIT to run or do other cardio exercises, women with PCOS might find more success by doing HIIT body weight circuits. With HIIT body weight circuits, you will spend your high-intensity time doing as many reps as possible of one body weight work out (like pushups, lunges, or squats), rest, and then repeat with another type of exercise. The internet is full of suggestions for HIIT body weight workouts, so you never have to get bored doing the same five exercises over and over again.

Setting and Starting an Exercise Routine

Even when you know what to do, it can be hard to start exercising. Most of us just don't enjoy it, and we always seem to have an excuse to skip a workout. How can you set and start an exercise routine that will really work for you?

First of all, fit your workout into your schedule, not the other way around. Trying to alter your life to fit your new exercise routine is stressful and makes it more difficult to develop a habit. Look at your current schedule and see where you could fit in a quick workout, even if it's just 20 minutes. Yes, you may have to sacrifice some TV time (or find a way to work out while watching TV!), but most women will be able to find at least a little wiggle room in their daily schedule to fit in a short workout. Working out from home saves you the trouble of traveling to a gym, and if you focus on body weight exercises, you don't need any fancy equipment to get started.

Mark on your calendar the days you want to work out, and try setting an alarm so you can't forget! After setting aside some time to exercise, spend at least a week using that time to simply take a walk around your neighborhood. It's easy, it gets you moving, and it starts ingraining in you the habit of exercise. After a week or two of walking at the scheduled times, you can swap out a one or two walks per week with HIIT strength training, and build from there. Don't feel like you need to do HIIT every day; it is a very intense form of exercise, and your body needs time to rest between workouts. You should have at least one day of recovery each week.

Recovery days don't have to be lethargic. A walk, some stretching, or playing around with your kids in the backyard are all fine activities for recovery days. Just listen to your body (your muscles will probably be screaming at you!) and take it easy; don't push yourself too hard.

Finally, if you are still struggling to stick to an exercise schedule, you might need to consider a different form of exercise. If you can find a workout you actually enjoy, you really boost your chances of success. If you hate traditional exercise programs, consider the following alternatives:

- Take a Zumba class, or try an instructional video at home
- Spend some time doing laps at the local public swimming pool
- Try martial arts like Kung Fu, Tae Kwon Do, Karate, or Capoeira
- Go hardcore with parkour (but be careful!)
- Find a gym that teaches adult gymnastics
- See if there's an indoor rock-climbing gym in your area

You've Started Exercising...Now Keep It Up!

Getting started with a workout routine is half the battle. The other half is maintaining that routine. It's so easy to go on vacation, get sick, or miss a few sessions and then never get back to your usual exercise schedule. When you have PCOS, it can be even harder to maintain your routine if, like many women, you suffer from chronic fatigue. If you aren't seeing quick results, it's easy to be discouraged and give up, as well.

This is where your list of goals, the one you came up with in section 2, comes in handy. Put that list up somewhere visible, where you can look at it every day when you're trying to talk yourself out of exercising. Remember the reasons why you started this program, the benefits to your health and your life – that's the best motivation to keep going.

Even the most motivated of us, though, will miss a workout now and then. If you're too fatigued to work out one day, ask yourself if you can manage just a short walk around the block, instead. And even if that's too much for you, that's okay; just dedicate yourself to resting up so that you'll be ready for the next scheduled workout. Missing a day is not the end of the world. Some people have a tendency to be too hard on themselves, and to feel like a failure after one bad day (or one bad week!), but that attitude is self-defeating. It's much better to focus on the future and on how you can succeed next time.

And what is the best way to succeed when you feel like giving up? Discipline.

Discipline takes motivation and will-power out of the equation, and while it's not always the most pleasant thing in the world, it can get you moving on those tough days when nothing else can. Planning ahead can be a big help towards becoming more disciplined. If you work out first thing in the morning, make sure to set out your clothes the night before. Get any equipment, towels, or videos ready before you go to bed, so that in the morning, all you have to do is get up and go.

If you work out in the evenings, or on your lunch hour at work, avoid distractions by letting your friends, family, and co-workers know what your schedule is. Let them know that it is important for you to have this time set aside for exercise; hopefully, they will support you by not asking you to schedule other activities during your workout time.

Finally, reward yourself! After meeting goals, even small ones, give yourself a reward that will reinforce your good habits. This doesn't mean splurging on an entire cheesecake because you met your goal weight. Choose rewards that will encourage you to continue working towards better health, like:

- Buy a new exercise outfit
- Treat yourself to a massage for those sore muscles
- Buy a fun video game that keeps you active (think "Dance, Dance, Revolution")
- Sign up for a fun class at a local gym

By reminding yourself of your motivation, practicing discipline, and encouraging good habits through positive reinforcement, you can succeed at building a life-long exercise habit!

Exercising is not just important for your physical health. It can also help your emotional and mental health, which, as we'll see next, is something important for women with PCOS to consider.

Step 6: Don't Let PCOS Play Mind Games

Many studies have proven that women with PCOS are more likely to suffer feelings of depression and anxiety, and are more likely to be diagnosed with a major psychiatric disorder. At least 60% of women with PCOS have at least one mental health problem. Generalized Anxiety Disorder, Major Depressive Disorder, and eating disorders are all more common in women with PCOS than in the general population. Taking care of yourself physically when you have PCOS is important, but it is just as vital to care of your mental health.

How PCOS Can Get Inside Your Head

Maybe it seems like an obvious link: obesity, excessive facial hair, and thinning hair on the head lead to women who are more stressed, have low self-esteem, and suffer from social anxiety. But worry over appearances is only one factor involved in the relationship between PCOS and mental health.

PCOS patients who are not overweight have the same risk for anxiety, depression, and eating disorders as obese PCOS patients. Regardless of outward appearances, women with PCOS tend to experience greater feelings of insecurity, fear of intimacy, and discomfort with introspection. It is possible that some of these emotional disturbances are caused by the imbalance of hormones experienced by women with PCOS. But, social factors do play a role as well.

We are all molded by our culture and environment to have a particular view of femininity. PCOS tends to challenge those views. Testosterone is what makes a man a man, right? But what if you're a women with high levels of testosterone, and the "manly" attributes (like facial hair) that come along with it?

And of course, whether a culture expresses it outright or not, having children is almost always considered an important part of being a woman. Yet, thousands of women with PCOS have been told they cannot have children, or they have been trying but have not been able to get pregnant. Feeling unfeminine because of having polycystic ovary syndrome has lead to many women developing anxiety, depression, and eating disorders.

Because of all this, it is extremely important for women with PCOS to take care of themselves emotionally, as well as physically.

Ways to Take Care of Your Mind

If you needed extra motivation to start exercising, this is it. A 2014 study published in *BMC Women's Health* assessed differences in depression between women with PCOS who exercised and ones who did not. It found that women who exercised showed fewer and more mild depression symptoms. The article concluded that "being more active may offer mental health benefits in managing PCOS." Taking a walk in the evening can help you sleep better, which is an added bonus!

MBSR (Mindfulness-Based Stress Reduction), also known as **mindful meditation**, has also been shown to help women with PCOS to reduce stress and anxiety. Participating in a program or class devoted to MBSR may prove helpful for you if you have never tried mindful meditation before. The basic principle is to focus on the present moment, observing one's body and surroundings mindfully, rather than allowing oneself to dwell on anxieties or negative thoughts. It can be a challenge when you first start out, but the effects of MBSR last far longer than the time spent meditating.

There are tons of other ways to de-stress: get a good night's sleep, enjoy the sunshine to get lots of vitamin D, listen to music, talk to friends and family. But before you can do any of that, you need to spend some time on introspection and evaluate what you need. Take time to take care of yourself! And if things get too hard to be fixed all on your own, don't be afraid to ask for professional help.

Add Another Doctor to Your Team

In section 2, we discussed specialists for PCOS like endocrinologists and gynecologists. But there is another specialist that many women with PCOS see as a routine part of their health care—a psychiatrist. Because PCOS comes with such a high risk for mood disorders and other mental health problems, it is definitely wise to be assessed by a professional from time to time.

There is a difference between experiencing stress and anxiety, which happens to everyone from time to time, and experiencing an anxiety disorder or other mental health disorder. The difference lies in the severity of the problem, and a psychiatrist is the best person to determine whether you need medication or other medical treatment to take care of your mental health. If you aren't sure whether or not you are ready or need to see a psychiatrist, talk to your primary care doctor. They should be able to give you a questionnaire that will help evaluate your depression/anxiety symptoms. Questions that might be asked include:

- Over the last two weeks, have you experienced:
    - Little or no interest in doing things
    - Feeling down, depressed, or hopeless
    - Having little energy or feeling tired all the time
    - Feeling like a failure, or like you've let down those you love
    - Trouble concentrating
    - Thoughts of harming yourself
    - Thoughts that you would be better off dead
    - Have these problems interfered with your work, social, or personal life?

There are many other questions that you will likely be asked – a psychiatric consultation usually lasts at least one hour – so be prepared to talk about your recent feelings, sleep and eating habits, as well as physical symptoms. It sounds scary, but for many women with PCOS, having a mental health specialist on their "team" is an invaluable support.

All the doctors in the world, however, cannot make up for the emotional support and motivation that family and friends can give you. That's why, in the last section of this book, we will talk about how to create a good support system of friends, family, and more.

Step 7: Create a Support Network

As individualized as PCOS is, it cannot be tackled alone. A support network consisting of family, friends, and doctors can help you with everything from deciding on treatment options to staying motivated to work out. However, due to the nature of this condition, many women hesitate to reach out to others for support. Many feel uncomfortable even mentioning PCOS, because they are afraid it will lead to awkward conversations (which is understandable; you don't want to talk about your irregular periods with just anyone). But there is a way to reach out while maintaining your privacy, and it all begins with how you approach the subject with friends and family.

Talking to Friends and Family About PCOS

So, by this point, you know all about your condition: how it works, what it means for you, how to manage it. It's time to share that information with friends and family. As you confront the inevitable highs and lows of living with PCOS, it will be nice to have someone on your side who understands and can provide emotional support. Of course, you don't need to feel pressured to share more information than you feel comfortable with. Your body and your health is your business. So how do you broach the subject while maintaining your privacy?

Be honest. You can explain that PCOS is a condition which disrupts the normal production of hormones. If more questions arise that you don't know the answer to, or feel embarrassed discussing, you can always answer, "I don't know," or "That's personal."

When you think about discussing your condition with friends and family, remember: the most important thing for your friends and family will not necessarily be technical explanations or symptom review; rather, their focus will likely be on your feelings. Are you scared? Insecure? Depressed? Let your family and friends know, and let them help you through those feelings. That's their best role as part of your support team. Technical and medical questions have other outlets.

Online Support Groups for Women with PCOS

As loving as friends and family are, sometimes you just need to talk with someone who knows exactly what you're going through. Having a group of fellow "cysters," either online or locally, can be a great outlet when you're feeling like "no one understands," or when you're wondering what sort of side effects to expect from a new treatment. Aside from numerous Facebook groups and groups within general fitness sites, here are a few specific PCOS support groups to check out.

myPCOSteam.com – My PCOS Team labels itself as "the social network for women diagnosed with

PCOS." Once you sign up, you can locate women in your area with PCOS, or you can search for users around the world to connect with who have similar symptoms or treatments.

Soulcysters.com – A combination of blogs, recipes, and stories – plus a message board with over 90,000 cysters to talk with.

PCOSchallenge.org – Since 2009, PCOS Challenge has been providing education and support to women with PCOS through online and offline programs, including a TV show and radio program.

Sign up with one of these groups, or another one, and spend some time looking around. It's truly amazing to see so many women speaking honestly and openly about things like balding, hot flashes, insecurity, and sadness. More than that, it's incredible to see how women respond to one another, encouraging and building one another up, recognizing that we're all in this together.

Making Local Connections

After signing up with one or more online support group, it will be easy to make local connections with other women who have PCOS. Remember that PCOS affects around 1 in 10 women, so there are probably a lot more "cysters" in your area than you might imagine. The local knowledge of restaurants, gyms, and stores that these local support groups provide helps give you even more precise, practical knowledge about how to treat your PCOS.

You may also be able to find support groups through local hospitals, medical groups, or insurance programs. Ask your doctors for suggestions; if there are any organized local support groups, PCOS specialists are likely to know about them.

Between family, friends, online and local support groups, you will have all the resources you need to help you through both the emotional and physical battles with PCOS.

Conclusion

As you continue your fight with PCOS, always remember the key steps outlined in this book:

1. Learn about and understand PCOS
2. Create a team of doctors who are knowledgeable about your condition
3. Define your goals and priorities, and let them guide your treatments
4. Pay attention to your nutrition, and eat foods that help regulate hormones
5. Create and stick to a regular exercise programs
6. Pay attention to your emotional and mental well-being
7. Create a network of people that can help support your journey

Polycystic ovary syndrome is not a disease; it's a condition, which is defined as "the circumstances affecting the way in which people live or work." PCOS will always affect the way we live and work, since there is no cure. But it does not *define* our lives or our work. Most importantly, it does not define our worth.

Don't let PCOS control your life; control your PCOS so that you can get on with your life!

Glossary of PCOS Symptoms and Treatments

Acanthosis Nigricans – This condition causes a darkening of patches of skin, and is usually related to insulin resistance or being overweight.

Acne – Due to imbalanced hormones, many adult women with PCOS struggle with acne. Androgen-promoting foods like dairy products can aggravate acne.

Amenorrhea – The absence of periods is called amenorrhea. A woman is considered to have amenorrhea if she has gone three or more months without having a period.

Anovulation – Anovulation is when a woman does not ovulate. Like amenorrhea, anovulation is usually considered to be three or more months without ovulation.

Bariatric Surgery – Lap-band (LABG) or BPD/DS are two types of bariatric surgery intended to help obese patients lose weight. A BMI of over 35 is considered obese. Bariatric surgery limits the amount of calories that a body can physically absorb. The recovery time for bariatric surgery is minimal; most patients are out of the hospital within 24 hours and back to work within one week.

Birth Control Pills – These contraceptives may be used to help regulate menstrual cycles and balance hormone levels. There are two classes of BCP;

Combination (Estrogen and Progestin) pills, and Progestin-only pills. Progestin is a synthetic version of progesterone, so both types of pill work by regulating the hormones associated with menstruation. Combination birth control pills include Levonorgestrel/Ethinyl estradiol and Norethindrone/Ethinyl estradiol. Progestin-only pills include Norgestrel, Norgestimate, Levonorgestrel, and Medroxyprogesterone. Side effects of birth control pills can include nausea, mood swings, weight gain, and (rarely) blood clotting or stroke.

Choriogonadotropin Alfa Injection - More commonly known as Ovidrel, this is a fertility treatment that stimulates ovulation. It is a hormone created from recombinant DNA. Common side effects include irritation at the injection site, nausea, vomiting, and abdominal pain. Rare but serious side effects include ovarian hyper-stimulation syndrome, ovarian enlargement, and blood clots.

Chronic Fatigue – Many women with PCOS suffer from chronic fatigue, or low energy.

Clomiphene – The brand name of Clomiphene is Clomid. It is a common fertility drug used to stimulate ovulation. Side effects can include breast tenderness, headache, abnormal uterine bleeding, blurred vision, nausea, and in rare cases, ovarian enlargement.

Cyst – A cyst is a fluid-filled sac. When talking about ovarian cysts, they can be inside the ovary, on the follicle where eggs are formed, or outside on the ovarian wall.

Cyst Aspiration – If ovarian cysts are present, and cause a great deal of pain, cyst aspiration can be performed to destroy the cysts. This procedure is very short, and performed in a doctor's office with local anesthetic. During the procedure, a needle is inserted through the vaginal wall and removes fluids from the cyst, which causes the cyst to collapse.

D&C (Dilation & Curettage) – For women with PCOS, D&C is used to treat heavy bleeding and potentially can improve chances for pregnancy. It is a procedure done in an office setting, usually by a gynecologist, with local anesthetic. During the procedure, the doctor will open the cervix, insert a tube or a spoon-shaped instrument, and scrape the inside of the uterus. While the procedure only takes a few minutes, the patient is usually kept in the office for a few hours to ensure that there are no post-surgical complications. Full recovery time can take at least one week.

Eflornithine – With a brand name of Vaniqa, Eflornithine is a prescribed medication used commonly to treat hirsutism. It comes as a cream, applied to the skin twice daily to inhibit hair growth. Common side effects include redness, rash, and stinging.

Electrolysis – Done by a professional called an electrologist, this is a permanent removal of unwanted hair by means of electrically destroying hair follicles. Usually, treatments are spread over several weeks. Immediate, temporary, side effects include swelling and redness of the affected area. In some cases, electrolysis may cause scarring or permanent skin discoloration.

Endometrial Ablation – For women with extremely heavy bleeding during menstruation, endometrial ablation can significantly reduce this symptom. The procedure can be done under general anesthetic in a hospital setting, or under local anesthetic in a doctor's office. Many different methods of ablation are used, but the end result is that the endometrium is destroyed, which leads to either a complete cessation of periods, or very light periods. Cramps, discharge, bleeding, and frequent urination are common in the week following an endometrial ablation. The procedure increases the risk for miscarriage and other problems during subsequent pregnancies, so it is not wise to have an endometrial ablation if you plan on getting pregnant any time in the future.

Endometrial Hyperplasia – When the uterine lining is exceedingly thick, it is called endometrial hyperplasia. Irregular or absent periods can cause endometrial hyperplasia. It is often treated with a D&C or with hormone replacement therapies to stimulate menstruation.

Endometriosis – When the endometrium, which usually lines the uterus, grows outside of the uterus, it is known as endometriosis. It is often very painful, and can cause cysts or scar tissue to develop. It is usually treated with hormone therapy or with surgery, depending on the severity.

Enlarged Ovaries – Cysts and endometriosis are common causes for enlarged ovaries. They can cause intense pain, heavy bleeding during menstruation, difficulty urinating, and other severe symptoms. Enlarged ovaries can also be an early sign of ovarian cancer, so it is important to see a doctor right away if you have symptoms of enlarge ovaries.

Finasteride – Finasteride is a prescription drug used to treat male-pattern baldness. Other names for this drug include Propecia and Proscar. It can be prescribed for women with PCOS who suffer from hair loss and hirsutism. For women, the common side effects of this drug include weight gain, breast tenderness, decreased libido, headache, and nausea. It can cause birth defects, so it is not recommended for women who are trying to get pregnant.

Follitropin Alfa for Injection – Commonly known as Gonal-F, this is an FDA-approved fertility treatment involving injections of a human follicle stimulating hormone which is derived from recombinant DNA. Side effects include cold symptoms, headache, rash, and irritation at the injection site. Rare but serious side effects include ovarian hyper-stimulation syndrome and ovarian enlargement.

Hirsutism – Hirsutism is a term meaning excessive hair growth, especially in a "male pattern," around the face, chest, and legs.

Hyperandrogenism – One of the primary symptoms of PCOS, hyperandrogenism means an excess of androgen, which are male hormones like testosterone.

Hysterectomy – A hysterectomy is a surgery which removes the uterus, and may include removing the ovaries (oophorectomy) and the cervix. A hysterectomy is often thought of as the final resort for women with severe PCOS symptoms, like heavy bleeding and cramping, who have not found success with any other treatments. However, it is *not* a cure for PCOS. It is a major surgery which may require up to six weeks of recovery time. It causes surgical menopause, meaning that a woman undergoing a hysterectomy will not be able to have children, will experience menopausal symptoms, and will likely need to be placed on hormone replacement therapy.

Inflammation – In the world of PCOS, the word inflammation is usually used in reference to chronic internal inflammation, which is a contributing cause of many serious diseases including metabolic syndrome, diabetes, and cancer. In a 2015 study called *The Role of Inflammation and Oxidative Stress in the Pathogenesis of Polycystic Ovary Syndrome,* researchers determined that inflammation is a contributing factor of anovulation in women with PCOS. There are many "Anti-Inflammatory" diets available which are meant to counteract the negative effects of inflammation.

IUD – Intra-Uterine Devices (IUD's) are a form of birth control which is inserted into the uterus by a doctor. They are long-acting, and do not carry the same risk of blood clotting and stroke that birth control pills have, because the hormones are absorbed directly into the uterus rather than traveling from the stomach via the blood stream. Risks involved with IUD use include infections, vaginal pain, and an increased risk of ectopic pregnancy.

Insulin Resistance – This is a condition where insulin is less effective at controlling blood sugar, leading to high blood sugar levels; if untreated, insulin resistance may lead to Type 2 Diabetes. It is very common in women with PCOS to have insulin resistance.

Leptin Resistance – Leptin is a hormone which regulates metabolism and appetite. Leptin resistance is a condition in which the body does not respond to leptin properly, causing a slow metabolism, increased hunger, and weight gain. Diet and exercise are the best treatments for leptin resistance.

Letrozole – Also known by the brand name Femera, Letrozole is a drug used to treat breast cancer in post-menopausal women. It has been used to treat fertility in women with PCOS, although this is an "off-label" use (not approved by the FDA). Common side effects include headache, dizziness, joint pain, edema, increased sweating, and feeling flushed. A rare but more serious side effect is a decrease in bone mineral density, so DEXA scans are often used to monitor women on Femera.

Leuprolide Acetate – Also called Lupron Depot, Leuprolide Acetate for depot suspension is a treatment for fibroid tumors and endometriosis. It can be used as part of a woman's fertility treatment if she has PCOS. It is a synthetic hormone which suppresses ovarian activity, and it can cause menopausal symptoms in some women. More rare, but serious, side effects include blood clots, vision problems, and convulsions.

Levothyroxine – Levothroid and Levoxyl are brand names for Levothyroxine, a synthetic thyroid hormone used to treat hypothyroidism. Common side effects include headache, fatigue, nervousness, moodiness, flushed skin, vomiting, diarrhea, abdominal cramps, muscle tremors, weakness, fast heartbeat, oligomenorrhea, and infertility. The most serious (though rare) side effects include seizures and decreased bone mineral density.

Liraglutide – Going by the brand name of Victoza, this drug is an injection which is sometimes prescribed for Type-2 Diabetes. While not an FDA-approved use, it is also sometimes used for PCOS to help with weight loss. It is a self-administered injection. Common side effects of Victoza include headache, nausea, diarrhea, and vomiting. More serious, but rare, side effects include thyroid cancer and pancreatitis.

Male-Pattern Baldness – Some women with PCOS suffer from what is commonly called "male-pattern" baldness, which is where hair loss happens on the crown of the head and along the hair line.

Menotropins for Injection – Repronex, or Menotropins for Injection, is a fertility medication which is a combination of hormones used to stimulate follicles in the ovaries. Common side effects include headache, dizziness, nausea, drowsiness, diarrhea, vomiting, fever, chills, shortness of breath, weakness, rash, muscle pain, and ovarian enlargement. Rare but serious side effects include ovarian hyper-stimulation syndrome and severe pulmonary conditions.

Metformin – Metformin is a prescription medication which has many brand names, including Glucophage, Glumetza, and Riomet. It is FDA-approved for use with patients who have Type-2 diabetes, but is commonly used as a treatment for PCOS. For women with PCOS, Metformin is known to help lower insulin resistance, promote weight loss, and can help promote fertility and regular menstruation. It is most effective when used in combination with diet and lifestyle changes. The most common side effect for Metformin is nausea.

Miscarriage – Women with PCOS have a greater likelihood of miscarriage when pregnant.

Obesity – Obesity is common for women with PCOS. Medically, a person is considered obese if their BMI is 35 or higher.

Oligomenorrhea – Irregular periods are called oligomenorrhea.

Oligovulation – Irregular ovulation is known as oligovulation.

Oophorectomy – A surgical procedure to remove the ovaries, oophorectomies may also be called ovariectomies. An oophorectomy causes permanent infertility and does not cure PCOS, but it is sometimes used as a treatment for severe cases of PCOS where the woman has not responded to other treatments. The procedure, recovery time, and risk factors are similar to that of a hysterectomy.

Ovarian Drilling – This surgery is performed in a hospital setting under general anesthesia. It is used to restore regular periods and promote fertility in women whose ovaries have a thickened surface due to PCOS. During ovarian drilling, a surgeon will make several tiny holes in the ovaries using a laser or electrosurgical knife, which helps decrease testosterone production. Women undergoing ovarian drilling can usually leave the hospital the same day, and are fully recovered in about two weeks. About 50% of women who undergo ovarian drilling are able to become pregnant in the first year after having the surgery.

Ovarian Hyper-stimulation Syndrome – OHSS causes a swelling of the ovaries and leaks fluid into the body. Many fertility treatments come with a risk of developing OHSS.

Paleo – The Paleo diet is popularly considered a treatment for PCOS; its basic principles include eating only natural, whole foods, and eating a diet high in protein and low in carbohydrates.

Sleep Apnea – When sleeping, a person with sleep apnea will stop breathing for short intervals, several times throughout the night. This is common in overweight individuals, including many women with PCOS. It can lead to excessive daytime sleepiness, chronic fatigue, as well as other health problems like high blood pressure. Sleep apnea is most often treated with a device known as a CPAP (Continuous Positive Airway Pressure) machine, which is worn while sleeping.

Spironolactone – Also known as Aldactone, this is a medication that some doctors will prescribe for acne or hirsutism, although this is not its FDA-approved use. Aldactone is typically used to treat high blood pressure, heart failure, and other cardiac conditions. Common side effects are headache, dizziness, rash, nausea, vomiting, and frequent urination. One rare, but serious, side effect is a severe electrolyte imbalance. Aldactone users are generally monitored with frequent blood work to prevent this issue.

About the Expert

Melissa Hayden is a writer, graphic designer, and cyster living near Seattle, Washington. She began her journey with PCOS when she was diagnosed at 18 years old. After dealing with many doctors, and feeling frustrated with the lack of personalized care, she has spent the last decade researching her condition and its many possible treatments. She is excited to be able to share that knowledge with others. You can join her "myPCOSteam" on mypcosteam.com/users/Ressa, or visit her professional website at sansseriffreelance.com.

HowExpert publishes quick 'how to' guides on all topics from A to Z by everyday experts. Visit HowExpert.com to learn more.

Recommended Resources

- <u>HowExpert.com</u> – Quick 'How To' Guides on All Topics from A to Z by Everyday Experts.
- <u>HowExpert.com/free</u> – Free HowExpert Email Newsletter.
- <u>HowExpert.com/books</u> – HowExpert Books
- <u>HowExpert.com/courses</u> – HowExpert Courses
- <u>HowExpert.com/clothing</u> – HowExpert Clothing
- <u>HowExpert.com/membership</u> – HowExpert Membership Site
- <u>HowExpert.com/affiliates</u> – HowExpert Affiliate Program
- <u>HowExpert.com/writers</u> – Write About Your #1 Passion/Knowledge/Expertise & Become a HowExpert Author.
- <u>HowExpert.com/resources</u> – Additional HowExpert Recommended Resources
- <u>YouTube.com/HowExpert</u> – Subscribe to HowExpert YouTube.
- <u>Instagram.com/HowExpert</u> – Follow HowExpert on Instagram.
- <u>Facebook.com/HowExpert</u> – Follow HowExpert on Facebook.

Printed by BoD™in Norderstedt, Germany